The Simple
Keto Diet Book

Delicious and Easy-Going
Recipes for Every Day incl.
Sides, Desserts and More

Michael A. Brown

ISBN - [9798837815522]

TABLE OF CONTENTS

Welcome and congratulations on starting a diet that can change your life for the better. Though we refer to Keto as a diet, it is a way of eating that can change your life and your health in many positive ways. The ketogenic diet, usually shortened to Keto, is a low-carb, high-fat diet known to help you lose weight and offer benefits when it comes to fighting against diabetes, epilepsy, cancer, and Alzheimer's disease. While some may have been on Keto for a while and just want some new recipe ideas, which this cookbook will offer, others may be new to Keto. To make sure you understand, we will provide the basics of Keto, plenty of recipes, a short meal plan, and more to help you get started.

Keto Basics

A Keto diet is low carb and high fat like some other diets. However, it involves a reduction in carbohydrate intake that is quite drastic, while replacing it with sources of fat. The reduction in carbohydrates in the diet sends the body into ketosis. When ketosis occurs, the body becomes efficient at using fat for energy and turning fat into ketones via the liver to supply energy for the brain. Ketogenic diets can significantly reduce blood sugar and insulin levels, but starting a new diet can be questionable if you have known health issues. Always check with your doctor before making any drastic dietary changes to ensure it is safe and progress can be tracked as needed.

Different Keto Diets

There are different versions of the ketogenic diet. It is up to you to decide which one is best for you and your lifestyle. The versions are shared below.

❖ Standard Ketogenic Diet – Very low, carb 10%, moderate protein 20%, and high fat 70%.

❖ Cyclical Ketogenic Diet – Higher carb refeeds, usually five ketogenic days followed by two days of high carbs

- ❖ Targeted Ketogenic Diet – Eating carbs only around workouts
- ❖ High Protein Ketogenic Diet – Much like the standards diet with5% carbs, 35% protein, and 60% fat

Both the standard and high protein ketogenic diets have been the focus of a great deal of research and are the most common. The targeted and cyclical versions are advanced and more extreme, usually reserved for athletes and bodybuilders.

Ketosis Defined

Ketosis is a medical term referring to a metabolic state in which the body uses fat instead of carbs for fuel. Ketosis happens when you are able to significantly reduce your carbohydrate intake and limit the body's supply of sugar (glucose), which is typically the main source of cell energy. Following a ketogenic diet is the most effective way to cause the body to enter ketosis. Most often, this means limiting carb intake to between 20 and 50 grams daily and instead filling up on fats found in meat, fish, nuts, eggs, and healthy oils. However, it is important to moderate protein consumption because protein, when consumed in high amounts, can be converted to glucose by the body. This can slow the ketosis transition. Practicing intermittent fasting can help you enter ketosis faster, with the most common method limiting food intake to about eight consecutive hours daily with 16 hours left for fasting. Though there are blood, urine, and breath tests to show whether you have entered ketosis, symptoms like frequent urination, increased thirst, dry mouth, and decreased hunger are also signals.

Research has shown that ketogenic diets are an effective way to lower risk factors for disease and lose weight. Some research has shown the Keto diet may be as effective as a low-fat diet. The Keto diet began as a tool used for treating neurological diseases, including epilepsy. However, further studies have shown that the diet can also be beneficial for other health conditions such as:

* ❖ Cancer
* ❖ Heart Disease
* ❖ Alzheimer's Disease
* ❖ Parkinson's Disease
* ❖ Epilepsy
* ❖ Brain Injuries
* ❖ Polycystic Ovary Syndrome

Though research into the benefits of Keto has shown promise in these areas, it is far from conclusive. Therefore, a diet should never be used in place of a doctor's orders, treatment, or medication without first discussing it with your doctor.

Foods to Avoid

As with any diet, there are foods to avoid while using the Keto diet. While numerous foods are acceptable, the list below explains what should be avoided or severely limited.

* ❖ High Carb Foods – Anything high in carbs should be avoided
* ❖ Sugary Foods – Foods such as fruit juice, soda, ice cream, candy, and cake should be avoided
* ❖ Fruit – All fruit except small portions of berries should be avoided
* ❖ Beans and Legumes – Beans and legumes such as peas, lentils, chickpeas, and kidney beans should be avoided
* ❖ Grains and Starches – Any wheat-based products, pasta, rice, and cereal should be avoided

- ❖ Root Vegetables and Tubers – Potatoes, including sweet potatoes, carrots, and parsnips, should be avoided
- ❖ Alcohol – Any form of alcohol should be avoided
- ❖ Condiments and Sauces – While some sauces are acceptable, those like barbecue sauce, teriyaki sauce, ketchup, and honey mustard should be avoided
- ❖ Unhealthy Fats – Fats like processed vegetable oils and mayonnaise should be avoided
- ❖ Low-Fat or Diet Products – Foods like sugar-free puddings, candy, desserts, and sweeteners, as well as low-fat salad dressings and condiments, should be avoided.

Foods to Enjoy

The list of foods to avoid may seem extensive, but there are still plenty of tasty foods to eat and prepare while on Keto. Some of these, most of which are included in the recipes in this book, are shared below.

- ❖ Meat – Steak, red meat, sausage, ham, bacon, turkey, and chicken
- ❖ Fatty Fish – Trout, mackerel, tuna, and salmon
- ❖ Eggs – Omega-3 whole eggs or pastured
- ❖ Cheese – Unprocessed cheeses like cream, cheddar, goat, mozzarella, or blue
- ❖ Butter and Cream – Heavy cream and grass-fed butter
- ❖ Healthy Oils – Coconut oil, extra virgin olive oil, or avocado oil
- ❖ Nuts and Seeds – Almonds, flaxseeds, walnuts, chia, or pumpkin
- ❖ Low Carb Vegetables – Tomatoes, peppers, green vegetables, or onions
- ❖ Condiments – Herbs, spices, salt, and pepper

Tips and Tricks

Getting started on the ketogenic diet can be a true challenge, so we wanted to include a few tips and tricks to familiarize yourself with before jumping into this new way of approaching food.

* ❖ Familiarize yourself with food labels, specifically the grams of fat, carbs, and fiber, to see how or if you can fit your favorite foods into the new diet.
* ❖ Plan out meals in advance to save time during the week and make sure ingredients are readily available. In addition, this helps curb snacking on the wrong types of food.
* ❖ Look into frozen Keto meals when under time constraints.
* ❖ When attending social gatherings, consider preparing and taking your own food to help you stick to your new diet.
* ❖ If eating out, choose meat or fish-based dish and replace high carb items with extra vegetables.
* ❖ For desserts, try berries with cream or a mixed cheese board.

Potential Side Effects

Generally, the ketogenic diet is safe for healthy people, but as the body adapts, you may have some side effects. Some people refer to this as the Keto flu, but these effects usually only last for a few days. The most common issues are constipation, vomiting, and diarrhea. Other, less common side effects include poor energy, foggy mental status, sleep issues, increased hunger, and decreased exercise performance. This can be minimized by trying a low-carb diet for a few weeks and then stepping up into Keto.

Additionally, a Keto diet can change the balance of minerals and water in the body. Add extra salt to meals and consider mineral supplements, such as MCT oil, creatine, whey, and even caffeine, to balance things out. Finally, as you start on a Keto diet, eat until you feel full without restricting calories too much.

Introduction

Now that you know the Keto basics, we can get started. In the pages of this cookbook, you will find recipes for breakfast, lunch, dinner, desserts, snacks, and extras. Also included is a sample meal plan and a section of FAQs for those new to Keto. Each recipe has the number of servings, carb, fat, and protein count included. Let's get started!

Breakfast

Start each morning with a good breakfast that will get your body working from the start. Whether you get to sit down with the family or need to grab something on the go, these recipes are simple and diverse while maintaining Keto guidelines.

Ham, Egg, Spinach, and Cheese Cups

Serves: 4 | Prep Time – 5 minutes | Cook Time – 15 minutes
Per Serving: Calories – 101 | Protein – 8 grams | Carbs – 1 gram | Fats – 7 grams

INGREDIENTS:

○ 4 Large Eggs
○ 3 Tbsp of Frozen spinach
○ 4 Small strips of thinly cut ham

○ 1 ½ Tbsp Cheddar cheese
○ Pinch of pepper and salt to taste

COOKING INSTRUCTIONS:

1 Preheat the oven to 400

2 Lightly fry the ham strips to set aside

3 Grease a muffin tray with oil or cooking spray and place the ham strips inside, folded on the bottom

4 Chop and dry spinach

5 Mix together all the eggs and beat in a bowl

6 Add spinach and mix well

7 Pour the spinach and egg mixture in the muffin tin over the ham (about ¾ of the way full)

8 Sprinkle cheese, salt, and pepper over each

9 Bake for 15 minutes or until the cheese has melted

Egg Muffin with Blackberry

Serves: 4 | Prep Time – 10 minutes | Cook Time – 15 minutes
Per Serving: Calories – 144 | Protein – 9 grams
| Carbs – 2 grams | Fats – 10 grams

INGREDIENTS:

- ○ 5 Large Eggs
- ○ 1 Tbsp Butter
- ○ 3 Tbsp Coconut flour
- ○ ½ C Fresh blackberries
- ○ 1 Tsp Ginger (grated)
- ○ ½ Tsp Vanilla
- ○ ½ Orange (zested)
- ○ 1 Tsp Rosemary (chopped finely)
- ○ ½ Tsp Salt (to flavor)

COOKING INSTRUCTIONS:

1   Preheat the oven to 350

2   In a blender, add eggs, butter, ginger, salt, vanilla, coconut flour, and orange zest to blend until well mixed

3   Once blended, add rosemary and blend again briefly

4   Pour the mixture into muffin cups (about ¾ full) and top each with a few blackberries

5   Bake for 15 minutes or until the eggs are set

Coconut Pancakes

Serves: 4 | Prep Time – 10 minutes | Cook Time – 8 minutes
Per Serving: Calories – 575 | Protein – 19 grams
| Carbs – 4 grams | Fats – 51 grams

INGREDIENTS:

- ○ 4 Large Eggs
- ○ 4 Oz Cream cheese
- ○ 2 Tbsp Almond flour
- ○ 8 Tbsp Maple syrup
- ○ 2 Tsp Cinnamon
- ○ 1 Tbsp Erythritol (sold at Walmart and Amazon in a bag, often in the baking section)
- ○ ½ C Shredded coconut

COOKING INSTRUCTIONS:

1 Put all the eggs in a bowl to beat well

2 Add the cream cheese and almond flour

3 Mix well

4 Add cinnamon, salt (to taste), and erythritol

5 Mix well

6 In a large frying pan on medium heat, pour four pancakes and fry on both sides until cooked to your preference

7 Remove from pan and sprinkle with shredded coconut and maple syrup

Frittata of Tofu

Serves: 4 | Prep Time – 15 minutes | Cook Time – 40 minutes
Per Serving: Calories – 347 | Protein – 22 grams
| Carbs – 7 grams | Fats – 24 grams

INGREDIENTS: ──────────────────────

- 24 Oz Extra-firm tofu (fully drained)
- 2 Tbsp Nutritional yeast
- ½ C Coconut flour
- 1 C Coconut milk (full-fat)
- 1 Tsp Curry powder
- 1 Green onion (diced)
- 1 Tsp Glucomannan powder (usually in pharmacy area with weight loss products)
- 1 C Button mushrooms (finely diced)
- ½ C Black olives (chopped)

COOKING INSTRUCTIONS:

1   Preheat the oven to 350

2   Line a medium casserole dish with parchment paper

3   In a food processor, combine tofu, nutritional yeast, coconut flour, coconut milk, glucomannan powder, curry, and salt and pepper to taste if needed

4   Process until smooth, then put the mixture into the casserole dish without spreading

5   Use a spoon to stir in mushrooms, olives, and green onion into the tofu mixture

6   Flatten the mixture into a casserole dish

7   Bake for 40 minutes or until the top is golden brown

8   After baking, cool for at least 5 minutes before slicing and serving

* If stored, place in airtight container and refrigerator for up to three days

Breakfast Casserole: Sausage and Egg

Serves: 4 | Prep Time – 20 minutes | Cook Time – 20-25 minutes
Per Serving: Calories – 295 | Protein – 20 grams
| Carbs – 2.5 grams | Fats – 22 grams

INGREDIENTS:

- ◯ 1 C Dark greens (kale, beet greens, or Swiss chard)
- ◯ 1 C Crumbled sausage (uncooked)
- ◯ 8 Medium Eggs or 6 large
- ◯ ½ C Parsley (rough chopped)
- ◯ 2 Tbsp Avocado oil

COOKING INSTRUCTIONS:

1 Preheat oven to 375

2 Slice greens into stems

3 Sauté in avocado oil over medium heat for several minutes

4 Add the sausage to the pan and continue to sauté until the sausage is almost fully cooked

5 Turn off the heat

6 Whisk eggs well in a bowl

7 Stir in kale, parsley, and sausage

8 Spray a baking pan (8x8) with avocado oil or wipe-on lightly

9 Pour mixture in a baking dish and bake until firm, top browning (20-25 minutes)

10 Allow to cool before cutting

Breakfast Doughnuts

Serves: 12 | Prep Time – 65 minutes | Cook Time – 25 minutes
Per Serving: Calories – 145 | Protein – 11 grams
| Carbs – 1 gram | Fats – 10 grams

INGREDIENTS:

- ○ 2 C Unsweetened almond milk
- ○ ½ Tsp Stevia powder
- ○ 4 Tbsp Coconut oil
- ○ 1 C Soy protein (organic and chocolate)
- ○ 1 C Almond flour
- ○ 1 Tsp Vanilla extract
- ○ 1 Tsp Glucomannan powder
- ○ 4 Tsp Cocoa powder

COOKING INSTRUCTIONS:

1 Preheat oven to 350

2 Use coconut oil to grease a donut pan for a dozen doughnuts

3 Use a mixing bowl to combine all ingredients and combine into a thick batter with a mixer or food processor

4 Ensure each doughnut ring is filled evenly

5 Bake for 25 minutes until the top of the doughnut is brown and a fork comes out clean

6 Remove doughnuts from the pan and cool for 30 minutes as they firm

7 Serve after firming

Western Scrambled Eggs

Serves: 6 | Prep Time – 5 minutes | Cook Time – 10 minutes
Per Serving: Calories – 239 | Protein – 14 grams |
Carbs – 2.4 grams | Fats – 19.3 grams

INGREDIENTS:

- 9 Large Eggs (beaten lightly)
- 3 Jalapenos (finely chopped)
- 2 Small diced tomatoes
- ¼ C Green onions (diced)
- 4 ½ Oz Cheddar cheese (shredded)
- 3 Tbsp Butter
- ¼ C Full cream milk

COOKING INSTRUCTIONS:

1   In a large skillet, over medium heat, melt the butter

2   Add tomatoes, green onions, and jalapenos to butter to cook for about 3 minutes, stir continually

3   In a bowl, whisk together eggs and cream, then pour into a skillet

4   Cook until eggs are almost set before adding cheese

5   Salt and pepper to taste

6   Cook until the cheese melts before serving

Cheese Egg Muffins

Serves: 6 | Prep Time – 10 minutes | Cook Time – 20 minutes
Per Serving: Calories – 144 | Protein – 8 grams |
Carbs – 1.5 grams | Fats – 12 grams

INGREDIENTS:

- ○ 4 Large Eggs
- ○ 2 Tbsp Greek yogurt (full fat)
- ○ 3 Tbsp Almond flour
- ○ ¼ Tsp Baking powder
- ○ 1 ½ C Parmesan cheese (shredded)

COOKING INSTRUCTIONS:

1   Preheat oven to 375
2   Combine yogurt and eggs in a bowl with salt and pepper to taste
3   Add flour and baking powder to egg mixture
4   Mix to form a smooth batter
5   Fold cheese into the mixture
6   Fill 6 silicone muffin cups with the mixture
7   Bake 20 minutes or until golden brown, turning the tray halfway through
8   Cool and serve

Avocado with Egg in Air Fryer

Serves: 8 | Prep Time – 15 minutes | Cook Time – 15 minutes
Per Serving: Calories – 223 | Protein – 8 grams |
Carbs – 4 grams | Fats – 12.6 grams

INGREDIENTS:

- 6 Medium Avocados (halved)
- 12 Eggs (medium or large)
- 2 Tsp Garlic powder
- 1 Tsp Sea salt
- ½ Tsp Black pepper (to taste)
- ½ C Parmesan cheese (shredded)

COOKING INSTRUCTIONS:

1. Preheat air fryer to 350
2. Halve avocados and scoop out 1/3 of each, place in a bowl
3. Put avocado halves in the air fryer face up and sprinkle lightly with salt and pepper to taste
4. Sprinkle with garlic powder before cracking eggs in avocado halves
5. Cook for 14 minutes in the air fryer
6. Serve

Beef and Fennel Hash in Air Fryer

Serves: 4 | Prep Time – 10 minutes | Cook Time – 20 minutes
Per Serving: Calories – 290 | Protein – 20 grams
| Carbs – 15 grams | Fats – 23 grams

INGREDIENTS:

- ❍ 4 C Ground beef
- ❍ 10 Large Mushrooms (sliced)
- ❍ 1 Onion (medium, sliced)
- ❍ 1 Tsp Smoked paprika
- ❍ 1 Avocado (large, diced)
- ❍ 4 Eggs (lightly beaten)
- ❍ 2 C Fresh fennel (chopped)
- ❍ Coconut oil for fryer

COOKING INSTRUCTIONS:

1 Preheat the air fryer to 375

2 Spray the air fryer pan with a small amount of coconut oil

3 Place mushrooms, onions, and salt and pepper to taste to the pan

4 Add uncooked ground beef, smoked paprika, and fennel to the pan

5 Crack eggs over the mixture and whisk gently

6 Cook for 20 minutes

7 Remove from pan and serve with fresh diced avocado

Easy Almond Crepes

Serves: 6 | Prep Time – 5 minutes | Cook Time – 10 minutes
Per Serving: Calories – 263 | Protein – 12.3 grams
| Carbs – 3 grams | | Fats – 23 grams

INGREDIENTS: ─────────────────────────

- ○ 12 Medium Eggs or 9 large eggs
- ○ ¾ C Unsweetened almond milk
- ○ 3 Tsp Almond flour
- ○ ½ C Parsley (finely chopped)
- ○ 6 Tbsp Coconut oil (used for frying)

COOKING INSTRUCTIONS: ──────────────

1 Combine all ingredients except coconut oil into a bowl and whisk until smooth

2 Let mixture stand uncovered for ten minutes to thicken slightly

3 Place a large skillet, greased with coconut oil, over medium heat until hot

4 Stir the batter and add a few tablespoons to the center of the skillet

5 Swirl skillet to thinly and evenly spread batter

6 Cook until golden brown (about two minutes)

7 Remove from skillet, fold lightly, and repeat for remaining batter

8 Serve while warm

Cinnamon French Toast in Air Fryer

Serves: 2 | Prep Time – 6 minutes | Cook Time – 8 minutes
Per Serving: Calories – 300 | Protein – 14 grams
| Carbs – 4.5 grams | Fats – 76 grams

INGREDIENTS:

- ◯ 4 Pieces of cinnamon swirl bread (large, homemade or store bought)
- ◯ 2 Tbsp Margarine
- ◯ 2 Eggs (large, beaten)
- ◯ 1 Tsp Nutmeg
- ◯ Ground cloves (to taste)

COOKING INSTRUCTIONS:

1 Preheat air fryer to 375

2 In a bowl, beat eggs with a pinch of salt and nutmeg to taste

3 Mix in cloves to taste

4 Butter both sides of the bread and cut into strips

5 Dredge bread strips in egg mixture and lay flat in the air fryer

6 Cook for two minutes

7 Still, in the fryer, spray both sides of bread with cooking spray and return for 4 more minutes or until browned lightly

8 Serve while warm

Lunch

The lunch recipes included are mostly quick prep meals or those that can be prepared ahead of time. Many can easily be prepared and taken to work to reheat as needed. Make sure you are not skipping meals on Keto, but only eating until you are full. Most lunches have multiple servings, so adjust as needed to fit the number of people you will be cooking for at the time.

Garlic Butter Shrimp

Serves: 4 | Prep Time – 10 minutes | Cook Time – 15 minutes
Per Serving: Calories – 329 | Protein – 32 grams
| Carbs – 5 grams | Fats – 20 grams

INGREDIENTS:

- ○ 6 Tsp Butter
- ○ 1 Pound Shrimp
- ○ 2 Lemons (halved)
- ○ 4 Garlic cloves (crushed)
- ○ ½ Tsp Red pepper flakes

COOKING INSTRUCTIONS:

1   Preheat oven to 425
2   Place butter in large baking pan and place in oven to melt
3   Sprinkle the shrimp with salt and pepper to taste
4   Slice one lemon in thin pieces and the other into wedges
5   Add the garlic and shrimp to the melted butter in the pan, place lemon slices on top, and sprinkle with pepper flakes
6   Bake for 15 minutes, stirring at the halfway point
7   Remove from oven and squeeze the juice from lemon wedges over the dish
8   Serve while warm

Turkey Milanese with a Crunch

Serves: 2 | Prep Time – 10 minutes | Cook Time – 10 minutes
Per Serving: Calories – 604 | Protein – 65 grams
| Carbs – 17 grams | Fats – 29 grams

INGREDIENTS:

- 2 Turkey breasts (skinless and boneless)
- 1 Egg (large)
- ½ C Coconut flour
- ½ C Bacon pieces (cooked, crushed)
- 2 Tbsp Olive oil
- ¼ Tsp Cayenne pepper
- Himalayan salt (to taste)

COOKING INSTRUCTIONS:

1   Pound out turkey breasts to ½ inch thick

2   On a small plate, mix coconut flour, cayenne pepper, and salt

3   On a second plate, lay out the crushed bacon bits

4   In a bowl, crack the egg and whisk slightly

5   Over medium heat, in a large skillet, heat olive oil until hot

6   Dredge turkey breasts in flour, then egg, and roll in bacon

7   Turn down heat to medium and put the turkey in the skillet until fully cooked (10 minutes)

8   Serve hot

Lasagna Keto Style

**Serves: 8 | Prep Time – 20 minutes | Cook Time – 30 minutes
Per Serving: Calories – 202 | Protein – 10 grams
| Carbs – 5 grams | Fats – 15 grams**

INGREDIENTS:

- ◯ 1 C Ground walnuts
- ◯ 3 C Marinara sauce
- ◯ ½ C Sundried tomatoes (chopped)
- ◯ 14 Oz Firm tofu (drained)
- ◯ ¼ C Basil (fresh preferred)
- ◯ 4 Tbsp Nutritional yeast (in most grocery stores with the spices)
- ◯ 1 ½ Tbsp Olive oil
- ◯ 2 Zucchinis (medium, thinly sliced lengthwise)

COOKING INSTRUCTIONS: ─────────────

1 Preheat the oven to 375

2 Blend walnuts, 1 C marinara, and tomatoes until smooth to create the walnut sauce

3 Set aside walnut sauce

4 With a clean blender, mix tofu, basil, nutritional yeast, and olive oil until smooth

5 Pour remaining marinara sauce in the bottom of a baking dish and cover with zucchini slices

6 Top with 1/3 of the tofu ricotta mixture and half the walnut sauce

7 Create another identical layer with zucchini slices, tofu ricotta, and walnut sauce

8 Top with remaining zucchini and tofu ricotta with salt and pepper to taste

9 Bake for 30-35 minutes

Keto Tofu Burgers

Serves: 4 | Prep Time – 35 minutes | Cook Time – 10 minutes
Per Serving: Calories – 321 | Protein – 11 grams
| Carbs – 6 grams | Fats – 28 grams

INGREDIENTS:

- ◯ 12 Oz Extra-firm tofu (drained)
- ◯ 1 C Coconut flour
- ◯ 2 Tbsp Soy sauce
- ◯ ½ C Sesame oil
- ◯ ½ C Coconut milk (full-fat)
- ◯ 2 Tbsp Rice vinegar
- ◯ ½ C Sesame seeds
- ◯ ½ C Cashews (crushed)
- ◯ ¼ C Nori flakes (often found in the international area of a local grocery store)

COOKING INSTRUCTIONS:

1 Preheat the oven to 400 and use parchment paper to line a baking tray

2 Press the tofu out to remove excess water and cut the block into 8 thin slices, set aside

3 Combine the soy sauce, sesame oil, coconut milk, and rice vinegar in a bowl, set aside

4 In another bowl, mix sesame seeds, cashews, and nori flakes

5 In a third bowl, pour the coconut flour

6 Take a slice of tofu and dip each side in flour, removing any extra, then dip it in the coconut milk mixture and finally coat it with the sesame seed mixture before placing it on the lined baking sheet

7 Repeat for all tofu slices

8 Bake for 10 minutes, flip, then bake an additional 10 minutes until both sides are crispy and browned

9 Remove and serve with a salad of greens if desired

Seared Tuna and Rice Bowl

Serves: 4 | Prep Time – 40 minutes | Cook Time – 10 minutes
Per Serving: Calories – 328 | Protein – 36 grams
| Carbs – 8 grams | Fats – 18 grams

INGREDIENTS:

- ⭘ 2 Tuna fillets (2 ounces with skin)
- ⭘ 8 Tbsp Soy sauce (divided)
- ⭘ 2 Tbsp Clarified butter (ghee if available)
- ⭘ 1 Cucumber (large)
- ⭘ 2 Avocados (diced)
- ⭘ 16 Oz Shirataki rice (available fresh and frozen in most grocery stores)

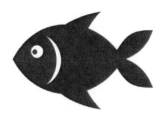

COOKING INSTRUCTIONS:

1. Place tuna in a baking dish with 6 Tbsp soy sauce
2. Cover and put in the refrigerator for at least 30 minutes
3. Slice cucumber thinly and cover in remaining soy sauce, set aside
4. In a skillet, over medium heat, melt butter (or ghee)
5. Add tuna, skin side down, to the skillet pouring a little of the marinade on top
6. Sear for 3-4 minutes on each side
7. Rinse rice in cold water and drain
8. Cook rice in boiling water for two minutes, drain
9. In a dry saucepan, dry roast rice over medium heat until dry and opaque
10. Remove skin from tuna fillets and cut tuna into small pieces
11. Season the diced avocado to taste
12. In four small bowls, layer rice, cucumbers, avocado, and tuna

Creamy Scallops

Serves: 4 | Prep Time – 5 minutes | Cook Time – 20 minutes
Per Serving: Calories – 782 | Protein – 24 grams
| Carbs – 11 grams | Fats – 73 grams

INGREDIENTS:

- ⭕ 8 Slices Turkey bacon
- ⭕ 2 C Heavy whipping cream
- ⭕ ½ C Parmesan cheese (grated)
- ⭕ 4 Tbsp Clarified butter
- ⭕ 16 Sea scallops (large, rinsed and patted dry)

COOKING INSTRUCTIONS: ───────────────

1   In a skillet over medium-high heat, cook turkey bacon until crisp

2   Move bacon to a paper towel covered plate to drain, but leave bacon grease

3   Lower heat to medium

4   Add cream, half of the butter, and cheese to grease

5   Season with salt and pepper to taste

6   Reduce to low and cook while constantly stirring until thickened (about ten minutes)

7   In a separate skillet over medium heat, melt the remaining butter until it is sizzling

8   Season scallops with salt and pepper to taste and place in skillet, cook 1 minute per side

9   Transfer scallops to a paper towel-lined plate

10 Divide the cream sauce between 4 plates, crumble bacon equally on top, and top with scallops

11 Serve immediately

Chicken Wings with Garlic Parmesan

**Serves: 2 | Prep Time – 10 minutes | Cook Time – 3 hours
Per Serving: Calories – 738 | Protein – 39 grams
| Carbs – 4 grams | Fats – 66 grams**

INGREDIENTS:

- ❍ 2 Pounds Chicken wings (fresh or frozen)
- ❍ 4 Cloves Garlic (finely chopped)
- ❍ ½ C Coconut aminos (in a bottle-also called coconut amino sauce)
- ❍ 1 Tbsp Fish sauce
- ❍ 2 Tbsp Sesame oil

COOKING INSTRUCTIONS:

1 Drain and pat dry chicken wings in a large bowl

2 In a small saucepan, over medium heat, heat garlic, coconut aminos, and fish sauce

3 Remove from heat and add sesame oil

4 Pour the mixture over wings and stir

5 Cool, then refrigerate covered overnight (stir occasionally)

6 Preheat oven to 375

7 Remove wings from marinade and place in a single layer on a baking sheet

8 Bake until cooked through

Grilled Turkey Skewers with Sauce

Serves: 4 | Prep Time – 70 minutes | Cook Time – 15 minutes
Per Serving: Calories – 586 | Protein – 75 grams
| Carbs – 15 grams | Fats – 29 grams

INGREDIENTS:

- ○ 2 Pounds Turkey breasts (boneless, skinless, and chunked)
- ○ 6 Tbsp Soy sauce
- ○ 1 ½ Tsp Siracha sauce
- ○ 6 Tsp Sesame oil
- ○ 4 Tbsp Peanut butter
- ○ Skewers

COOKING INSTRUCTIONS:

1. In a large sealable bag, combine turkey chunks, 4 Tbsp soy sauce, 1 Tsp siracha, and 4 Tsp sesame oil

2. Seal the bag, shake gently to coat, and let marinate in the refrigerator for at least an hour or up to overnight

3. If using wooden skewers, soak in water for 30 minutes before use

4. Preheat the grill to low with a grill pan or skillet warming as it preheats with a small bit of clarified butter allowed to melt

5. Thread turkey chunks onto skewers and cook over low for 10-15 minutes, flipping halfway through

6. For the dipping sauce: mix remaining soy sauce, sriracha, sesame oil, and peanut butter well to dip skewers

Chicken and Cheesy Broccoli

Serves: 4 | Prep Time – 10 minutes | Cook Time – 60 minutes
Per Serving: Calories – 935 | Protein – 75 grams
| Carbs – 10 grams | Fats – 66 grams

INGREDIENTS:

- ○ 4 Chicken breasts (boneless, skinless)
- ○ 8 Bacon slices
- ○ 12 Oz Cream cheese (room temp)
- ○ 4 C Frozen broccoli florets (thawed)
- ○ 1 C Cheddar cheese (shredded)

COOKING INSTRUCTIONS:

1 Preheat oven to 375

2 Using a large casserole dish, lightly coated with clarified butter, place seasoned (salt and pepper) chicken and bacon slices in the oven for 25 minutes

3 Remove from oven, but leave the oven on

4 Transfer the chicken to a cutting board and shred with a fork, season again to taste

5 Remove bacon from dish and place on a paper towel to crisp

6 Once the bacon has cooled and crisped, crumble

7 In a separate bowl, mix cream cheese, broccoli, chicken, and half the bacon

8 Pour and even out the mixture in the casserole dish

9 Top with shredded cheese and remaining bacon

10 Bake for 35 minutes until slightly browned and bubbling

Beef Roast with Parmesan

Serves: 4 | Prep Time – 10 minutes | Cook Time – 25 minutes
Per Serving: Calories – 370 | Protein – 40 grams
| Carbs – 6 grams | Fats – 21 grams

INGREDIENTS:

- ½ C Parmesan (grated)
- ½ C Pork rinds (crushed)
- 1 Beef roast (small, whole, or sliced)
- 1 Pound Asparagus spears
- 2 Tbsp Garlic powder (use to taste)
- Olive oil

COOKING INSTRUCTIONS:

1. Preheat oven to 350
2. Line a baking sheet with foil
3. Pat the roast dry
4. Mix pork rinds, parmesan, and garlic in a bowl
5. Roll roast in the mixture
6. Place on a baking sheet and drizzle lightly with olive oil
7. Place asparagus around the roast and drizzle with oil
8. Sprinkle leftover pork rind mixture on asparagus
9. Bake for 20-25 minutes or until cooked through
10. Serve hot

Dinner

Dinner recipes are family-friendly and created to share. A variety of common foods are combined in unique ways to maintain the Keto diet while still enjoying tasty food. Remember to vary your food choices each day, so the diet does not get boring.

Air Fryer Ham Wrapped Shrimp

Serves: 4 | Prep Time – 10 minutes | Cook Time – 10 minutes
Per Serving: Calories – 276 | Protein – 26 grams
| Carbs – 2 grams | Fats – 18 grams

INGREDIENTS:

- ⭘ 8 Oz Shrimp
- ⭘ 5 Oz Ham (sliced thin)
- ⭘ 1 Tsp Lemon juice (fresh)
- ⭘ ½ Tsp Salt
- ⭘ ½ Tsp Turmeric
- ⭘ ½ Tsp Rosemary (dried)
- ⭘ ½ Tsp Canola oil

COOKING INSTRUCTIONS:

1 Peel all shrimp before sprinkling with lemon juice and salt to taste

2 Mix well with hands to coat all shrimp

3 Mix rosemary and turmeric, then sprinkle on shrimp

4 Wrap each shrimp in a slice of ham, securing with a toothpick

5 Preheat the air fryer to 360 and spray with canola oil lightly

6 Cook shrimp for five minutes for each side

7 Let cool before serving

Pork Stuffed Peppers

Serves: 4 | Prep Time – 10 minutes | Cook Time – 20 minutes
Per Serving: Calories – 707 | Protein – 40 grams
| Carbs – 22 grams | Fats – 52 grams

INGREDIENTS:

- ❍ 1 Pound Ground pork
- ❍ 6 Bell peppers (large)
- ❍ ½ C Sour cream
- ❍ 2 Avocados (large)
- ❍ 1 C Shredded cheese (your choice)
- ❍ Clarified butter

COOKING INSTRUCTIONS:

1   Preheat oven to 400

2   Line a baking sheet with foil

3   Melt just enough clarified butter to cover the bottom of a skillet

4   When the butter has melted and is warm, add pork, and season to taste with salt and pepper

5   Break up and cook until lightly browned

6   Prepare peppers by cutting off the top and then slicing in half; remove seeds and ribs

7   Place peppers on the pan and fill with cooked pork and sprinkle with cheese

8   Bake for 10 minutes

9   In a separate bowl, mix avocado and sour cream until well blended

10 Serve stuffed peppers with a dollop of avocado crema

Skirt Steak with Chimichurri

Serves: 2 | Prep Time – 12 hours | Cook Time – 10 minutes
Per Serving: Calories – 718 | Protein – 70 grams
| Carbs – 22 grams | Fats – 46 grams

INGREDIENTS:

- ¼ C Soy sauce
- ¼ C Chimichurri sauce
- 1 Tbsp Vinegar (apple cider)
- ½ C Olive oil
- 1 Pound Skirt steak
- Clarified butter

COOKING INSTRUCTIONS:

1 Combine all ingredients except chimichurri sauce in a plastic, sealable bag, shake lightly, and leave to marinate in the refrigerator overnight

2 Remove steak and lightly dry with a paper towel, then season to taste

3 Melt a small amount of clarified butter over high heat in a skillet

4 Once melted, brown steak on both sides

5 Rest steak at least five minutes before slicing

6 Top with chimichurri sauce

Skillet Tofu

Serves: 4 | Prep Time – 15 minutes | Cook Time – 15 minutes
Per Serving: Calories – 311 | Protein – 18 grams
| Carbs – 7 grams | Fats – 24 grams

INGREDIENTS:

- ❍ 24 Oz Extra firm tofu (drained, cubed)
- ❍ 4 Garlic cloves
- ❍ 4 Tbsp Coconut oil
- ❍ 2 Onions (medium, chopped)
- ❍ 4 Red chilis (finely chopped)
- ❍ 4 Tbsp Maple syrup (low carb)
- ❍ 1 Tbsp Mustard
- ❍ ½ C Water

COOKING INSTRUCTIONS:

1 In a large skillet over medium heat, melt coconut oil and brown tofu lightly

2 In a blender, mix garlic, onions, syrup, soy sauce, and mustard into a paste

3 Add the paste to skillet until it begins to caramelize

4 Turn down to medium and slowly add water

5 Let cook, occasionally stirring until most of the water has evaporated

6 Remove from heat

7 Allow to cool slightly before serving

Turkey Quesadilla

Serves: 4 | Prep Time – 5 minutes | Cook Time – 5 minutes
Per Serving: Calories – 414 | Protein – 29 grams
| Carbs – 20 grams | Fats – 35 grams

INGREDIENTS:

- ○ 2 Tbsp Olive oil
- ○ 4 Tortillas (large, low-carb)
- ○ 1 C Shredded cheese (Mexican or cheddar)
- ○ 4 Tbsp Sour cream
- ○ Tajin seasoning (with Mexican seasonings in-store)
- ○ 4 Oz Turkey (cooked, shredded)

COOKING INSTRUCTIONS:

1   Over medium heat, heat olive oil in a large skillet

2   Place one tortilla down, top with cheese, turkey, and Tajin to taste)

3   Top with the second tortilla

4   After bottom browns slightly, flip and brown the other side (about 1-2 minutes per side)

5   Repeat for each quesadilla

6   Slice quesadilla and top with sour cream

7   Serve hot

BBQ Ribs

**Serves: 4 | Prep Time – 10 minutes | Cook Time – 4 hours
Per Serving: Calories – 956 | Protein – 68 grams
| Carbs – 5 grams | Fats – 72 grams**

INGREDIENTS:

- ○ 2 Pound Pork ribs
- ○ Himalayan salt
- ○ Ground black pepper
- ○ 2.5 Oz Dry rib seasoning pack
- ○ 1 C BBQ sauce (sugar-free)

COOKING INSTRUCTIONS:

1 Preheat the crockpot to high

2 Season ribs with salt, pepper, and seasoning rub

3 Place the ribs, bone side inward, along sides of the cooker

4 Pour sauce on both sides of ribs, just enough to coat

5 Cover and cook for 4 hours until tender

Bibimbap with Steak

Serves: 4 | Prep Time – 10 minutes | Cook Time – 15 minutes
Per Serving: Calories – 261 | Protein – 21 grams
| Carbs – 3 grams | Fats – 18 grams

INGREDIENTS:

- ○ 2 Tbsp Clarified butter
- ○ 1 Pound Ground beef
- ○ 2 Eggs (medium)
- ○ ¼ C Scallions (chopped finely)
- ○ 2 Garlic cloves (mashed)
- ○ Ginger (optional, to taste)
- ○ 2 Pound Cauliflower (frozen, riced, thawed)
- ○ 2 C Peas and Carrots (frozen)
- ○ Red pepper flakes
- ○ 1 Tsp Sugar
- ○ 1 Tsp Sesame oil
- ○ 1 Tsp Rice vinegar
- ○ Himalayan salt
- ○ Black pepper
- ○ 5 Tbsp Soy sauce

COOKING INSTRUCTIONS:

1 In a large skillet over medium-high heat, melt butter and brown ground beef seasoned to taste

2 After browning, stir in half of the soy sauce and lower to medium heat

3 In a separate skillet, scramble two eggs and put them in a bowl

4 Sauté scallions, garlic, and ginger until softened

5 Add cauliflower rice, sugar, red pepper flakes, and soy sauce to taste

6 Heat over medium for about 3 minutes, stirring continuously

7 Add thawed peas and carrots and heat until vegetables are warm, rice is tender

8 Stir in rice vinegar, sesame oil, and eggs

9 Mix rice and vegetables with pork and split between four bowls

10 Serve hot

Burgers with Siracha Mayo

Serves: 2 | Prep Time – 10 minutes | Cook Time – 10 minutes
Per Serving: Calories – 575 | Protein – 31 grams
| Carbs – 2 grams | Fats – 49 grams

INGREDIENTS:

- ○ 12 Oz Ground beef
- ○ 2 Scallions (medium, entire scallion sliced thinly)
- ○ 1 Tsp Sesame oil
- ○ 2 Tbsp Mayonnaise
- ○ 1 Tbsp Sriracha sauce

COOKING INSTRUCTIONS:

1 Combine ground beef, scallions, and sesame oil with seasoning to taste

2 Form two evenly sized patties

3 Add a small amount of oil to a skillet over medium heat and allow to get hot

4 Cook burger on both sides to the desired temperature

5 In a small bowl, mix mayo and siracha well

6 Wrap burgers in a lettuce leaf or try one of the Keto-friendly breads in the snack section as a bun, top with a small bit of mayo mixture

Creamy Ranch Porkchops

Serves: 6 | Prep Time – 5 minutes | Cook Time – 25 minutes
Per Serving: Calories – 477 | Protein – 25 grams
| Carbs – 2 grams | Fats – 39 grams

INGREDIENTS:

- ○ 6 Pork chops (boneless, thick cut)
- ○ 8 Oz Cream cheese (full fat)
- ○ 8 Tbsp Salted butter
- ○ ½ C Heavy cream
- ○ ½ C Chicken broth
- ○ Sea salt
- ○ Black pepper
- ○ 3 Tbsp Ranch seasoning

COOKING INSTRUCTIONS:

1 Pat pork chops dry and sprinkle with salt and pepper to taste (both sides)

2 Heat butter over medium-high heat until melted in a skillet

3 Sear chops on each side until golden brown and cooked, reduce heat to medium

4 Remove pork chops

5 Pour chicken broth in the pan and scrape all browned bits together to deglaze

6 Mix in cream cheese, cream, and stir continuously until smooth

7 Add in ranch seasoning until fully combined

8 Reduce heat to low and put pork chops back in

9 Cover and simmer for 10 minutes

Creamy Garlic Chicken Soup

Serves: 4 | Prep Time – 10 minutes | Cook Time – 10 minutes
Per Serving: Calories – 307 | Protein – 18 grams
| Carbs – 2 grams | Fats – 25 grams

INGREDIENTS:

- 1 Pack Garlic and herb seasoning (found with other packaged seasonings)
- 2 Tbsp Clarified butter
- 1 Chicken breast (large)
- 4 Oz Cream cheese (cubed)
- 14.5 Oz Chicken broth
- ¼ C Heavy cream
- Salt (to taste)

COOKING INSTRUCTIONS:

1 Boil then shred chicken breast
2 In a saucepan, over medium heat, melt all butter
3 Add chicken to pan and coat with butter
4 As the chicken warms, add cream cheese and seasoning
5 Mix well
6 Once the cream cheese melts, add broth and heavy cream
7 Bring to a boil, then reduce heat to low to simmer for 3-4 minutes
8 Add salt if needed and serve

Zucchini Pasta with Garlic and Parmesan

Serves: 4 | Prep Time – 8 minutes | Cook Time – 12 minutes
Per Serving: Calories – 197 | Protein – 11 grams
| Carbs –11 grams | Fats – 14 grams

INGREDIENTS:

- ○ 4 Zucchinis (medium)
- ○ 3 Tbsp Olive oil (extra virgin)
- ○ 1 Tbsp garlic (minced)
- ○ ½ Tsp Red pepper flakes (adjust to taste)
- ○ 2 Tomatoes (chopped) or 12 Oz canned tomatoes
- ○ ½ C Parmesan cheese (shredded)
- ○ 1 C Basil leaves (torn into pieces)
- ○ 1 Tsp Cornstarch
- ○ 2 Tsp Cold water
- ○ Salt (to taste)

COOKING INSTRUCTIONS:

1. Trim and spiralize zucchini leaving the peel on and making extra-long noodles
2. In a deep skillet, add olive oil, garlic, and pepper flakes over medium heat
3. When the oil bubbles around the garlic, add zucchini noodles
4. Toss the noodles using tongs and cook to al dente (wilted with a crunch)
5. As the noodles cook, continue to toss to mix and get all evenly cooked
6. Stir in tomatoes, cheese, and basil and allow to cook for one minute
7. Transfer noodles, basil, and tomatoes to a serving dish, but leave the liquid
8. Bring the remaining liquid to a simmer
9. In a small bowl, combine water and cornstarch and whisk into the simmering liquid
10. Cook until thickened into a sauce (about a minute)
11. Pour over the noodles, top with extra parmesan
12. Serve

Cheesy Potato Casserole

Serves: 6 | Prep Time – 10 minutes | Cook Time – 65 minutes
Per Serving: Calories – 857 | Protein – 6 grams
| Carbs – 15 grams | Fats – 36 grams

INGREDIENTS:

- ⃝ 3 Pounds Yukon gold potatoes (peeled and quartered)
- ⃝ 30 Oz Package of frozen hash browns (thaw at least 20 minutes before)
- ⃝ ½ C Butter (melted, room temperature)
- ⃝ 1 Tsp Salt
- ⃝ 1 ½ C Cheddar cheese (shredded)
- ⃝ 2 C Sour cream or Greek yogurt
- ⃝ ½ C Whole milk
- ⃝ ½ Tsp Black pepper
- ⃝ ½ Tsp Paprika
- ⃝ ½ Tsp Garlic powder
- ⃝ 2 Tsp Thyme (dried)
- ⃝ 3 Tbsp Chives
- ⃝ 1 Can Cream of chicken soup
- ⃝ ½ Yellow onion (large, chopped)
- ⃝ 1 Clove Garlic (grated)
- ⃝ ½ C Fried onions (dried, crushed)
- ⃝ 2 C Cheese Doritos (crushed)

COOKING INSTRUCTIONS:

1   Preheat oven to 375

2   Over medium heat, in a frying pan, add 1 Tbsp of butter and onion, cooking until onion is soft (5 minutes)

3   In a mixing bowl, combine hash browns, salt, pepper, chives, sour cream, cheddar, cream of chicken, and onions; mix well

4   Put the mixture in a casserole dish

5   Cook in the oven for 30 minutes

6   Take the casserole out and stir well

7   Bake for another 20-30 minutes until the top and sides bubble

8   Remove from oven and add crushed fried onions and Doritos, bake for an additional 3-5 minutes without burning (optional)

9   Serve warm

Sausage Stuffed Mushrooms

Serves: 8 | Prep Time – 15 minutes | Cook Time – 25 minutes
Per Serving: Calories – 281 | Protein – 15 grams
| Carbs – 6 grams | Fats – 22 grams

INGREDIENTS:

- ❍ 1 Pound Cremini mushrooms
- ❍ 1 Pound Italian sausage
- ❍ 4 Oz Cream cheese
- ❍ ½ C Mozzarella (shredded)
- ❍ ½ Tsp Red pepper flakes
- ❍ ¼ C Parmesan (grated)
- ❍ Salt (to taste)

COOKING INSTRUCTIONS:

1   Preheat oven to 350
2   Clean the mushrooms and remove the stems
3   In a skillet over medium heat, brown the sausage
4   Once cooked, move to a heat-safe bowl
5   To the sausage, add cream cheese and mozzarella, stir well (add salt and red pepper to taste)
6   Spoon the sausage mixture into the mushroom caps
7   Sprinkle parmesan on top
8   Place in a casserole dish, single layer
9   Bake for 25 minutes until mushrooms are soft and cheese is browned

Broccoli Nuggets

Serves: 10 | Prep Time – 10 minutes | Cook Time – 30 minutes
Per Serving: Calories – 176 | Protein – 6 grams
| Carbs – 2 grams | Fats – 10 grams

INGREDIENTS:

- ○ 3 C Broccoli florets
- ○ ½ C Parmesan cheese (shredded)
- ○ 1/3 C Mexican blend cheese (shredded)
- ○ ½ C Flax meal
- ○ 2 Eggs (large)
- ○ ¼ C Nutritional yeast
- ○ ½ Tsp Ground turmeric
- ○ 1 Tsp Chicken base paste
- ○ ¼ Tsp Himalayan salt (to taste)
- ○ Pepper (to taste)
- ○ Olive oil and clarified butter (for cooking)

COOKING INSTRUCTIONS:

1 Cut broccoli and place in a blender until crumb fine

2 Mix broccoli, parmesan, and Mexican cheese in a bowl, set aside

3 In a blender, put eggs, flax meal, yeast, paste, salt, pepper, and turmeric and blend well (about 20 seconds)

4 Pour into broccoli and stir with a fork until the mixture becomes moist and loosely sticks together

5 In a cast-iron skillet, over medium heat, heat equal parts butter and oil

6 Form broccoli mixture into balls and 1.5 Tbsp in size and flatten

7 Place in a hot skillet

8 Cook in oil for 5-6 minutes, turning halfway through

9 Allow to cool before serving

10 Sugar-free ketchup can be used for dipping

Side Dishes

Keto does not stop with the main dish. On the following pages are recipes for side dishes that are Keto-friendly, easy to make, and paired with the dish of your choice. Get creative and work with ingredients you know well to create dishes of your own.

Broccoli Salad

Serves: 10 | Prep Time – 35 minutes | Cook Time – 10 minutes
Per Serving: Calories – 285 | Protein – 6 grams
| Carbs – 3 grams | Fats – 26 grams

INGREDIENTS:

- ○ 2 Heads Broccoli (tops only or florets that are precut and fresh)
- ○ 8 Slices Bacon (no sugar added, cooked, and crumbled)
- ○ 1 C Red onion (diced)
- ○ ½ C Sunflower seeds (roasted, salted)
- ○ 1 C Cheddar cheese (shredded)
- ○ 1 C Mayonnaise
- ○ 2 Tbsp Apple cider vinegar
- ○ 3 Tbsp Erythritol

COOKING INSTRUCTIONS:

1   In a small bowl, mix mayonnaise, erythritol, and vinegar set aside

2   Combine all remaining ingredients in a large bowl

3   Pour on dressing from step one

4   Mix well

5   Chill for at least one hour before serving

Loaded Roasted Radishes

Serves: 6 | Prep Time – 5 minutes | Cook Time – 40 minutes
Per Serving: Calories – 214 | Protein – 11 grams
| Carbs – 6 grams | Fats – 28 grams

INGREDIENTS:

- ○ 4 C Radishes (washed, trimmed, halved)
- ○ 1 ½ Tbsp Olive oil (extra virgin)
- ○ ½ Tsp Salt
- ○ ¼ Tsp Pepper
- ○ ½ C Colby jack cheese (shredded)
- ○ 8 Slices Bacon (cooked, crumbled)
- ○ 2 Green onions (finely chopped)
- ○ ½ C Keto ranch dressing (recipe included in "extras" section)

COOKING INSTRUCTIONS:

1   Preheat oven to 425

2   Place all the radishes in a bowl and toss with olive oil, salt, and pepper

3   Spread radishes in a single layer on a non-stick baking sheet

4   Bake until crisp-tender, about 35 minutes, stirring once while roasting

5   Once roasting is complete, sprinkle with cheese and place back in over to melt cheese

6   Remove from oven and drizzle with ranch, bacon, and green onions

Broccoli Mash

Serves: 8 | Prep Time – 5 minutes | Cook Time – 10 minutes
Per Serving: Calories – 225 | Protein – 2 grams
| Carbs – 27 grams | Fats – 22 grams

INGREDIENTS:

- ○ 4 C Broccoli florets (fresh or frozen)
- ○ 1 C Water
- ○ 1 Tsp Lemon juice
- ○ 2 ½ Tbsp Clarified butter (melted)
- ○ ½ Tsp Ginger paste
- ○ 1 Clove Garlic
- ○ Salt and pepper to taste
- ○ ½ C Gouda (grated)
- ○ 2 Tbsp Heavy cream
- ○ ½ Tbsp Coriander (crushed)
- ○ 1 Tsp Red pepper flakes (crushed)
- ○ 4 Sweet potatoes (peeled, diced)

COOKING INSTRUCTIONS:

1 Over medium heat, put all broccoli and sweet potatoes in water and leave for 5 minutes

2 Pour out the water and remove it from the heat

3 In a separate bowl, put broccoli and potatoes and top with lemon juice, ginger, garlic, butter, pepper flakes, salt, pepper, heavy cream, and cheese

4 Mix well

5 Using a potato masher or mixer, mash all ingredients

6 Add chopped coriander at the end, mix well before serving

Garlic Butter Mushrooms

Serves: 2 | Prep Time – 3 minutes | Cook Time – 20 minutes
Per Serving: Calories – 273 | Protein – 8 grams
| Carbs – 8 grams | Fats – 12 grams

INGREDIENTS:

- 1 Pound Button mushroom (small as possible or cut in half)
- 1 Tbsp Olive oil
- 4 Cloves Garlic (chopped finely)
- 1 Tsp Sea salt
- ¼ Tsp Pepper
- 3 Tbsp Clarified butter
- 2 Tbsp Parsley (chopped)

COOKING INSTRUCTIONS:

1 Over high heat, in a large frying pan, saute oil, garlic, salt, and pepper

2 Place mushrooms in the mixture to be coated well

3 Still over heat, continue stirring as you add butter 1 Tbsp at a time, allowing each coat to melt over mushrooms

4 When mushrooms start releasing liquid, reduce heat to medium and occasionally stir until liquid evaporates and mushrooms turn deep brown (10-15 minutes)

5 Remove from heat, mix in parsley, serve

Cauliflower Casserole

**Serves: 4 | Prep Time – 10 minutes | Cook Time – 10 minutes
Per Serving: Calories – 298 | Protein – 11 grams
| Carbs – 7.4 grams | Fats – 15 grams**

INGREDIENTS:

- ○ 1 Pound Cauliflower (the equivalent of a large head)
- ○ ½ C Sour cream
- ○ 1 C Cheddar cheese (grated)
- ○ ½ C Mayonnaise
- ○ 4 Slices Bacon (fried, crispy, crumbled)
- ○ 6 Tbsp Chives (fresh chopped)
- ○ 3 Tbsp Clarified butter
- ○ ¼ Tsp Garlic powder
- ○ Salt and pepper to taste

COOKING INSTRUCTIONS:

1 Begin by washing the cauliflower and cutting florets into small chunks

2 Place in a saucepan with 2 Tbsp of water to boil (more if needed) and cover on medium heat for 5-8 minutes until tender but not overcooked

3 Remove from heat and drain, rest for two minutes

4 Place all cauliflower in a food processor and mix until fluffy

5 Add garlic, butter, and sour cream to the processor

6 Mix until the consistency of mashed potatoes

7 Remove mixture and add chives, bacon, and cheddar cheese

8 Blend well

9 Season to taste

10 Put the whole dish in the oven or microwave to melt the cheese before serving

Bacon-Wrapped Jalapeno Poppers

Serves: 12 | Prep Time – 25 minutes | Cook Time – 25 minutes
Per Serving: Calories – 198 | Protein – 6 grams
| Carbs – 2 grams | Fats – 14 grams

INGREDIENTS:

- ○ 12 Jalapeno peppers (3-4 inches each)
- ○ 8 Oz Cream cheese (softened)
- ○ 1 C Cheddar cheese
- ○ ½ Tsp Onion powder
- ○ ½ Tsp Salt
- ○ ½ Tsp Pepper
- ○ 12 Slices Bacon
- ○ Cooking spray of choice

COOKING INSTRUCTIONS: ───────────────

1 Preheat oven to 400

2 Line a sheet pan with foil and coat the foil with cooking spray to prevent sticking

3 Cut jalapenos in half lengthwise, removing all ribs and seeds

4 In a bowl, mix cream cheese, cheddar, salt, pepper, and onion powder

5 Once combined, fill each jalapeno half with the cheese mixture

6 Cut all bacon slices in half lengthwise

7 Wrap each pepper in a slice of bacon and secure it with a toothpick while cooking

8 Place peppers on the baking sheet, single layer, and bake for 20-25 minutes until bacon is browned

9 Serve immediately for best results

Coleslaw (with Mayonnaise) Dressing

Serves: 10 | Prep Time – 5 minutes | Cook Time – 7 minutes
Per Serving: Calories – 300 | Protein – 2 grams |
Carbs – 9.2 grams | Fats – 37 grams

INGREDIENTS:

- ❍ 2 Pounds cabbage (red or green)
- ❍ 3 Carrots (large)
- ❍ 1 ½ C Dressing (recipe below)
- ❍ 1 C Mayonnaise
- ❍ ¼ C Apple cider vinegar or white wine
- ❍ 1 Tbsp Sugar (powered)
- ❍ ½ Tsp Salt

* Dressing can also be made from sour cream or buttermilk. These recipes are in the extra section.

COOKING INSTRUCTIONS:

1   Shred the cabbage in 2-3 inch pieces and shred further in a food processor

2   Place in a large bowl and set aside

3   Peel the carrots and shred them in the processor

4   Mix carrots into the cabbage

5   In a small bowl, mix all the dressing ingredients well with a whisk

6   Pour the dressing over the cabbage and toss gently to combine

7   Refrigerate for at least one hour before serving to build flavor

Zucchini Fries (Air Fryer)

Serves: 4 | Prep Time – 10 minutes | Cook Time – 25 minutes
Per Serving: Calories – 117 | Protein – 7 grams
| Carbs – 5 grams | Fats – 8 grams

INGREDIENTS:

- ⭕ 2 Zucchinis (medium)
- ⭕ 1 Egg (large, beaten)
- ⭕ 1/3 C Almond flour
- ⭕ ½ C Parmesan cheese (grated)
- ⭕ 1 Tsp Italian seasoning
- ⭕ ½ Tsp Garlic powder
- ⭕ ¼ Tsp Sea salt (to taste)
- ⭕ ¼ Tsp Black pepper (to taste)
- ⭕ Cooking spray

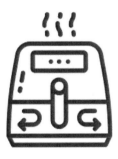

COOKING INSTRUCTIONS:

1   Slice each zucchini in half and then into sticks (about ½ inch thick and 3-4 inches long)

2   In a bowl, mix flour, cheese, seasoning, garlic powder, salt, and pepper; mix well

3   Whisk egg until well beaten

4   Dredge each stick in the egg, then roll in dry ingredients

5   Repeat for all sticks

6   Spray sticks with cooking spray

7   For air fryer: place fries in a single layer and fry at 400 for 10 minutes or until crisp

8   For oven: On a lined pan, place fries in a single layer, bake at 425 for 18-22 minutes, flipping halfway through

Green Bean Casserole

Serves: 8 | Prep Time – 15 minutes | Cook Time – 30 minutes
Per Serving: Calories – 243 | Protein – 15 grams |
Carbs –6 grams | Fats – 6 grams

INGREDIENTS:

- ○ 4 C Green beans (fresh or frozen)
- ○ 2 ½ Tbsp Stick butter
- ○ ½ C Diced onions
- ○ ½ C Cream or half and half
- ○ 1 Tsp Soy sauce
- ○ ½ C Mushrooms (fresh)
- ○ 2 Cloves Garlic (minced)
- ○ 1 Tsp Worcestershire sauce
- ○ 3 C Chicken broth (optional)
- ○ 10.5 Oz Cream of mushroom soup (canned)
- ○ ½ C Crispy fried onions
- ○ 1 C Cheddar (grated)
- ○ Salt and pepper to taste

COOKING INSTRUCTIONS: ———————————————

1   Preheat oven to 350

2   In a large pot over medium-high heat, boil 2 quarts of salted water

3   Once boiling, add beans to water for 5 minutes

4   After boiling, drain and remove from heat, set aside

5   In a large skillet, melt the butter over medium heat and then use the skillet to sauté the onions and mushrooms together until softened (2-3 minutes)

6   Mix in fresh garlic and cook another minute

7   Add chicken broth or mushroom soup and mix in the green beans in the sauce

8   Cook 10 minutes, then reduce heat to medium-low

9   Season with salt and pepper to taste

10   Add cheese and stir in cream, and cook until it thickens (4-5 minutes)

11   Remove from heat and stir well

12   Pour in a casserole dish

13   Top with crispy onions and bake for 10 minutes or until browned

14   Serve hot

15   If desired, add bacon crumbles or jalapenos for a bit of variety

Stuffing

Serves: 4 | Prep Time – 10 minutes | Cook Time – 10 minutes
Per Serving: Calories – 127 | Protein – 4.3 grams
| Carbs – 8 grams | Fats – 9 grams

INGREDIENTS:

- ○ 4 Slices Keto bread or rolls (store-bought or homemade) * homemade recipe under extras
- ○ 3 Tbsp Clarified butter (melted)
- ○ 2 Stalks Celery (chopped)
- ○ ¼ C Leeks (chopped)
- ○ ½ Tsp Garlic (minced)
- ○ 1 Tsp Italian blend seasoning
- ○ ¼ Tsp Sage
- ○ ½ Tsp Salt and pepper (to taste)
- ○ Olive oil
- ○ ½ C Chicken broth

COOKING INSTRUCTIONS:

1 Preheat oven to 350

2 Crumble Keto bread and drizzle with olive oil

3 Bake for 5 minutes until lightly browned

4 Sauté chopped vegetables in olive oil for two minutes

5 Mix all together with melted butter and chicken broth

6 Bake in a dish, foil-covered, for 10 minutes, uncover and bake for 5

7 Serve warm

Desserts

Whether dessert is special for certain occasions or something you enjoy nightly, these simple recipes will satisfy you. Many can be prepared and stored for days or even months. A few require no cooking at all. So, whether you are craving fruit, chocolate, or something unique, these recipes will fulfill your wishes.

Coconut and Chocolate Popsicles

Serves: 4 | Prep Time – 2 hours | Cook Time – 0 minutes
Per Serving: Calories – 193 | Protein – 2 grams
| Carbs – 2 grams | Fats – 20 grams

INGREDIENTS:

- ½ Can (13.5 Oz) Coconut cream
- 2 Tsp Stevia
- 2 Tsp Unsweetened cocoa powder
- 2 Tbsp Chocolate chips (sugar-free)

COOKING INSTRUCTIONS:

1 Mix coconut cream, sweetener, and cocoa powder in a blender

2 Pour into popsicle molds, dropping in chocolate chips

3 Freeze at least two hours

Keto-Friendly Cheesecake Bites

Serves: 4 | Prep Time – 3 hours | Cook Time – 30 minutes
Per Serving: Calories – 169 | Protein – 5 grams
| Carbs – 9 grams | Fats – 15 grams

INGREDIENTS:

- ○ 4 Oz Cream cheese (room temperature)
- ○ ¼ C Sour cream
- ○ 2 Eggs (large)
- ○ 5 ½ Tbsp Stevia
- ○ ¼ Tsp Vanilla extract

COOKING INSTRUCTIONS:

1   Preheat oven to 350

2   Mix all ingredients with a hand mixer until well blended

3   Place liners in a muffin tin and evenly pour cheesecake batter

4   Bake 30 minutes

5   Refrigerate until cool (3 hours) before serving

Chocolate Chip Bread with Macadamia Nut Butter

Serves: 4 | Prep Time – 75 minutes | Cook Time – 18 minutes
Per Serving: Calories – 202 | Protein – 5 grams
| Carbs – 3 grams | Fats – 15 grams

INGREDIENTS:

- ○ 1 C Macadamia butter (instructions included)
- ○ 2 C Macadamia nuts
- ○ ¼ C Coconut flour
- ○ ½ C Chocolate chips
- ○ ½ Tsp Baking soda
- ○ ½ Tsp Baking powder
- ○ 2 Tbsp Maple syrup
- ○ 2 Tsp Apple cider vinegar
- ○ 1 Tbsp Vanilla extract

COOKING INSTRUCTIONS:

1 Begin by making the macadamia butter (any extra can be stored in the refrigerator)

2 Place macadamia nuts in a bowl and cover with water, leave to absorb for an hour

3 Rinse nuts well and blend in a food processor until a creamy consistency

4 Preheat oven to 350

5 Place 1 C of macadamia butter in a bowl

6 In the food processor, blend eggs, baking powder, baking soda, vanilla, coconut flour, and vinegar until smooth

7 Add chocolate chips and butter and mix well with a spoon

8 Pour the batter into a loaf pan, tapping out bubbles

9 Bake for 30 minutes

Coconut Cinnamon Bread

Serves: 10 | Prep Time – 15 minutes | Cook Time – 30 minutes
Per Serving: Calories – 80 | Protein – 2 grams
| Carbs – 16 grams | Fats – 1 gram

INGREDIENTS:

- ○ 3 Eggs (large)
- ○ 1 Tsp Vinegar
- ○ 3 Tbsp Butter (salted)
- ○ 1 Tsp Cinnamon
- ○ 2 Tbsp Water
- ○ ½ C Coconut flour
- ○ ½ Tsp Baking soda
- ○ ½ Tsp Baking powder
- ○ Greek yogurt
- ○ Pinch of stevia (or sweetener of choice)

COOKING INSTRUCTIONS:

1 Preheat the oven to 350

2 Lightly oil the loaf pan and line the bottom with parchment paper

3 Mix all dry ingredients until well blended

4 Add all wet ingredients and mix well

5 Taste for sweetness level and adjust with more sweetener if needed

6 Let stand for 3 minutes and mix well again

7 Spread batter in a loaf pan

8 Bake 25-30 minutes (until a toothpick comes out of center clean)

9 Cool on a wire rack, slice into ten slices

10 Store extras in the refrigerator

Mini Cream Doughnut

Serves: 8 | Prep Time – 15 minutes | Cook Time – 35 minutes
Per Serving: Calories – 319 | Protein – 10 grams
| Carbs – 3 grams | Fats – 17 grams

INGREDIENTS:

- ○ 3 Eggs (large)
- ○ 3 Oz Cream cheese
- ○ 1 Tsp Baking powder
- ○ 1 Tsp Vanilla extract
- ○ 4 Tsp Erythritol extract (found on Amazon as "Keto Flavor Pack")
- ○ 1 Tbsp + 2 Tsp Coconut flour
- ○ 10 Drops stevia (liquid)
- ○ 3 Tbsp + 2 Tsp Almond flour

COOKING INSTRUCTIONS:

1 Blend all ingredients thoroughly in an immersion blender

2 Spray a preheated doughnut maker with coconut oil

3 Pour the batter equally into the mold and cook for 3 minutes per side

4 Remove and allow to cool

5 Repeat with remaining batter

Chocolate Mousse

Serves: 4 | Prep Time – 35 minutes | Cook Time – 10 minutes
Per Serving: Calories – 218 | Protein – 2 grams
| Carbs – 5 grams | Fats – 23 grams

INGREDIENTS:

- ○ 1 C Heavy whipping cream
- ○ ¼ C Cocoa powder (unsweetened, sifted)
- ○ ¼ C Powdered sweetener (your choice)
- ○ 1 Tsp Vanilla extract
- ○ ¼ Tsp Salt (kosher)

COOKING INSTRUCTIONS:

1   Whisk whipping cream into stiff peaks

2   Add cocoa, sweetener, vanilla, and salt to whipped cream

3   Mix again

4   Serve

Keto-Friendly Chocolate Cake with Whipped Cream Icing

Serves: 9 | Prep Time – 35 minutes | Cook Time – 10 minutes
Per Serving: Calories – 358 | Protein – 8 grams
| Carbs – 11 grams | Fats – 33 grams

INGREDIENTS: ───────────────────────

Cake:

- ○ ¾ C Coconut flour
- ○ ¾ C Stevia or swerve
- ○ ½ C Cocoa powder
- ○ 6 Eggs (large)
- ○ 2 Tsp Baking powder
- ○ ½ C Melted butter
- ○ 2/3 C Heavy whipping cream

Icing:

- ○ 1 C Heavy whipping cream
- ○ ¼ C Stevia or swerve
- ○ 1 Tsp Vanilla extract
- ○ 1/3 C Cocoa powder (sifted)

COOKING INSTRUCTIONS:

1 Preheat oven to 350

2 Grease an 8x8 cake pan

3 In a mixer, combine and mix all ingredients well

4 Pour the batter evenly into the cake pan

5 Bake 25 minutes or until center springs back when touched

6 Let cool completely before icing

7 Whip whipping cream to stiff peaks in a mixer

8 Add sweetener, cocoa powder, and vanilla and continue mixing until combined

9 Use icing to ice cake and serve

10 Leftovers should be refrigerated

Chocolate Chip Cookies

Serves: 21 | Prep Time – 10 minutes | Cook Time – 12 minutes
Per Serving: Calories – 179 | Protein – 5 grams
| Carbs – 4 grams | Fats – 17 grams

INGREDIENTS:

- ○ 2 Eggs (large)
- ○ 2 Tsp Vanilla extract
- ○ 3 C Almond flour
- ○ ¾ C Softened butter or coconut oil
- ○ 2/3 C Swerve sweetener
- ○ ½ Tsp Baking soda
- ○ ½ Tsp Salt (kosher)
- ○ 4.5 Oz Chocolate chips (sugar-free)

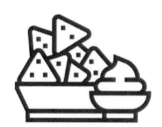

COOKING INSTRUCTIONS: —————————————————

1   Preheat oven to 350

2   Using a mixer, combine softened butter and swerve

3   Add in eggs and vanilla while continuing to mix

4   In a separate bowl, mix dry ingredients, except chocolate chips, until combined

5   Combine wet and dry ingredients and mix as chocolate chips are folded in

6   Using a cookie scoop, scoop 21 cookies onto a lined baking sheet

7   Press slightly to flatten

8   Bake for 10-12 minutes

9   Let cool and eat

10 Will stay fresh in an airtight container for up to 4 days or can refrigerate and then freeze for up to three months

Blueberry Crisp

Serves: 2 | Prep Time – 5 minutes | Cook Time – 20 minutes
Per Serving: Calories – 390 | Protein – 6 grams
| Carbs – 17 grams | Fats – 35 grams

INGREDIENTS: ────────────────

- ❍ 1 C Blueberries (fresh or frozen)
- ❍ ¼ C Pecan halves (optional)
- ❍ 2 Tbsp Salted butter
- ❍ 2 Tbsp Swerve
- ❍ 1 Tbsp Ground flax
- ❍ 2 Tbsp Heavy cream
- ❍ 1/8 C Almond flour
- ❍ ½ Tsp Cinnamon
- ❍ ½ Tsp Vanilla extract
- ❍ ¼ Tsp Salt (kosher)

COOKING INSTRUCTIONS: ────────────

1   Preheat oven to 400

2   In 1 C oven-safe ramekins, combine ½ C blueberries, and ½ Tbsp swerve

3   In a food processor, combine pecans, almond flour, remaining swerve, butter, vanilla, cinnamon, flax, and salt, pulse until combined

4   Spread mixture on top of blueberries

5   Place ramekins on a baking sheet in the center of the oven for 15-20 minutes until the top is brown

6   Serve with heavy cream drizzled on top

Chocolate, Almond, Bacon Bark

Serves: 8 | Prep Time – 30 minutes | Cook Time – 0 minutes
Per Serving: Calories – 157 | Protein – 4 grams
| Carbs – 13 grams | Fats – 13 grams

INGREDIENTS:

- ○ 9 Oz Chocolate chips (sugar-free)
- ○ 2 Slices Bacon (cooked and crumbled)
- ○ ½ C Almonds (chopped)

COOKING INSTRUCTIONS:

1. Melt chocolate chips in a double boiler or microwave (in a microwave-safe bowl, heat 30 seconds, stir, heat 30 seconds, stir, heat 15 seconds, stir)
2. Add almonds to melted chocolate, stir
3. Line a baking sheet with parchment paper
4. Pour the chocolate mixture on the parchment in a thin layer
5. Sprinkle bacon on top and press lightly with a spatula
6. Refrigerate for 20 minutes or until chocolate hardens
7. Separate from parchment paper and break into 8 pieces

Snacks

If you happen to get hungry between meals, several Keto-friendly options can get you to the next meal. Though a few recipes are included, most are just easy-to-grab snacks that can be eaten on the go.

- Cheese – cheddar, blue, mozzarella, and goat are the best options
- Nuts or Seeds – one handful at a time
- Olives – 10 to 12 total
- Egg – hardboiled or deviled
- Greek Yogurt – 1 C, full fat, mixed with a Tbsp of nut butter or Tsp of cocoa powder
- Keto-friendly Snack Bars – Recipe below
- Keto Sushi Bites – Recipe below

Keto-Friendly Snack Bars

Serves: 18 | Prep Time – 4 minutes | Cook Time – 1 minute
Per Serving: Calories – 139 | Protein – 9 grams
| Carbs – 5 grams | Fats – 10 grams

INGREDIENTS:

- 1 4/5 C Smooth almond butter
- ½ C Sweetener of choice (honey, sugar-free maple syrup, or agave nectar)
- 2/3 C Coconut flour
- 1 4/5 Tbsp Almond flour
- 1 4/5 C Chocolate chips (optional)

COOKING INSTRUCTIONS:

1 Put muffin liners in a mini muffin pan and set them aside

2 In a large bowl, add all ingredients and mix well (if the batter is too thick, add syrup or sweetener to form a batter, thick but pourable)

3 Melt chocolate on a double boiler

4 Fill each muffin tin evenly until all batter is used, cover each with a bit of melted chocolate

5 Refrigerate until firm

Sushi Bites

Serves: 4 | Prep Time – 15 minutes | Cook Time – 0 minutes
Per Serving: Calories – 165 | Protein – 17 grams
| Carbs – 3 grams | Fats – 12 grams

INGREDIENTS:

- ○ 6 Oz Sushi-grade tuna or salmon
- ○ 1 Pack Nori seaweed sheets
- ○ 2 Avocados (optional)
- ○ 1 Bell pepper (optional)
- ○ 1 Cucumber (large)
- ○ 1 Oz Cream cheese

* Choose the raw vegetables you most enjoy or choose all vegetables instead of fish

COOKING INSTRUCTIONS:

1   Lay out four sheets of nori seaweed on a flat, dry surface

2   Evenly chop up all vegetables and fish

3   Spread cream cheese on nori lightly

4   Fill with fish and vegetables

5   Lightly wet nori edges and roll tightly

6   Slice or eat as a wrap

Extras

Sometimes, we all need a dipping sauce, some variety, or even a bit of bread. The few recipes in this section will help you create a few of those extras that may be missing from other recipes or meals.

Keto Ranch Dressing

Serves: 12 | Prep Time – 12 minutes | Cook Time – 0 minutes
Per Serving: Calories – 123 | Protein – 1 grams
| Carbs – 1 gram | Fats – 13 grams

INGREDIENTS:

- ○ ¾ C Mayonnaise
- ○ ¼ C Sour cream
- ○ Unsweetened almond milk (as needed)
- ○ Salt and pepper (as needed)
- ○ 1 ½ Tbsp Dried parsley
- ○ 2 Tsp Dried dill weed
- ○ ¼ Tsp Onion powder
- ○ ¼ Tsp Garlic powder
- ○ ½ Tsp Swerve
- ○ 1 Tsp Worcestershire sauce (optional to taste)
- ○ ½ Tsp Apple cider vinegar
- ○ Keto buttermilk (see below)
- ○ ¼ C Heavy whipping cream
- ○ ¾ Tsp Apple cider vinegar

COOKING INSTRUCTIONS:

1   Begin by making the Keto buttermilk

2   In a bowl, mix whipping cream and vinegar well

3   Wait 6-8 minutes, stir once or twice between, until the consistency of buttermilk

4   In a separate bowl, mix dry ingredients for the dressing

5   In the buttermilk bowl, mix all wet ingredients except almond milk

6   Combine all ingredients and mix well

7   If dressing is too thick, add almond milk as needed

8   Ready to eat immediately, but is best served after overnight refrigeration

Dressing – Sour Cream

Serves: 5 | Prep Time – 2 minutes | Cook Time – 0 minutes
Per Serving: Calories – 30 | Protein – 0.5 grams
| Carbs – 1 gram | Fats – 5 grams

INGREDIENTS:

- ½ C Sour cream
- ½ C Mayonnaise
- ½ C Apple cider vinegar or white wine
- 1 Tbsp Sugar (powered)
- ½ Tsp Salt

COOKING INSTRUCTIONS:

1   Mix all ingredients and blend with a whisk
2   Store extra in the refrigerator

Dressing – Buttermilk

Serves: 5 | Prep Time – 5 minutes | Cook Time – 0 minutes
Per Serving: Calories – 100 | Protein – 1 gram |
Carbs – 2 grams | Fats – 18 grams

INGREDIENTS:

- ½ C Buttermilk
- ½ C Mayonnaise
- 1 Tbsp Sugar (powdered)
- ¼ C Apple cider vinegar
- ½ Tsp Salt

COOKING INSTRUCTIONS:

1   Mix all ingredients in a small bowl and blend with a whisk
2   Store extra in the refrigerator for up to three days

Garlic Knots

Serves: 8 | Prep Time – 25 minutes | Cook Time – 20 minutes
Per Serving: Calories – 220 | Protein – 7 grams
| Carbs – 5 grams | Fats – 19 grams

INGREDIENTS: ─────────────────────

- ○ ½ C Almond flour
- ○ ¼ C Coconut flour
- ○ 2 Tsp Baking powder
- ○ ½ Tsp Garlic powder
- ○ ¼ Tsp Salt
- ○ 1 ½ C Mozzarella cheese (shredded, part-skim)
- ○ 5 Tbsp Butter (melted)
- ○ 1 Egg (large)

Butter:

- ○ 3 Tbsp Butter (melted)
- ○ 2 Tbsp Parmesan (freshly grated)
- ○ 2 Tsp Garlic (minced)
- ○ ¾ Tsp Salt (kosher)
- ○ ½ Tsp Parsley (dried)

COOKING INSTRUCTIONS: ——————————————————

1   Preheat oven to 350

2   Line a baking sheet with parchment paper

3   In a bowl, combine almond and coconut flour, baking powder, salt, and garlic powder

4   In a saucepan, melt cheese over low heat until it can be mixed

5   Add butter and egg, stir well

6   Still, on low heat, stir in dry ingredients and stir until dough forms (some large sections of cheese will be seen)

7   Place dough on parchment paper and kneed until uniform

8   Divide the dough into 16 equal portions

9   Roll each into a 7-inch log and tie into a gentle knot

10 Place on parchment a few inches apart

11 In a separate bowl, mix ingredients for butter

12 Brush about half the butter over the knits before baking

13 Bake knots for 15-20 minutes until golden brown and firm to the touch

14 Remove from oven and brush with remaining butter

Fathead Rolls aka Keto Bread

Serves: 4 | Prep Time – 10 minutes | Cook Time – 15 minutes
Per Serving: Calories – 160 | Protein – 7 grams |
Carbs – 2.5 grams | Fats – 13 grams

INGREDIENTS:

- ○ 2 Oz Cream cheese
- ○ ¾ C Mozzarella (shredded)
- ○ 1 Egg (large)
- ○ ¼ Tsp Garlic powder
- ○ 1/3 C Almond flour
- ○ 2 Tsp Baking powder
- ○ ½ C Cheddar cheese (shredded)

COOKING INSTRUCTIONS:

1   Preheat oven to 425

2   In a microwave-safe bowl, mix cream cheese and mozzarella

3   Microwave for 20 seconds at a time, stir, then continue until melted

4   In a separate bowl, beat egg

5   Add dry ingredients to the egg, mix well

6   Work the Mozzarella and cream cheese mixture into the dough (will be sticky)

7   Add in cheddar cheese

8   Spoon dough onto plastic wrap

9   Dust top with almond flour

10 Fold the plastic over the dough and work into a ball gently

11 Cover and refrigerate for 30 minutes

12 Once chilled, cut dough into 4 pieces and roll each piece into a ball

13 Cut the ball in half to form a top and bottom bun

14 On a sheet pan lined with parchment paper, place cut side down

15 Bake 10-12 minutes until golden and set up

Sample Weekly Meal Plan

Breakfast	Lunch	Dinner	Side
Egg Muffin with Blackberry	Tofu Burger	Ranch Porkchops	Broccoli Mash
Ham, Egg, Spinach, Cheese Cup	Seared Tuna in Rice Bowl	Sausage Stuffed Mushrooms	Green Salad (Keto Ranch)
Avocado with Egg	Chicken Wings	Zucchini Pasta	Garlic Knots
Cinnamon French Toast	Cheesy Chicken Broccoli	Burgers with Siracha Mayo	Loaded Radishes
Sausage & Egg Casserole	Turkey Skewers	BBQ Ribs	Zucchini Fries

Keto Frequently Asked Questions

1. Is a Keto diet safe?

The Keto diet is considered safe in most circumstances. Before making any extreme dietary changes, it is best to consult your doctor, but generally, Keto is safe. The three known situations in which you need to make adaptations are diabetes, high blood pressure, or breastfeeding. If on medication for any condition, it is always best to speak to a doctor as well.

2. Is Keto safe for the kidneys?

Since the Keto diet has gained popularity over the years, many myths and concerns have been voiced. One of those concerns is whether this high-protein diet is safe for the kidneys. Keto is kidney safe because it is a high-fat diet with moderate protein levels, and if your kidneys are functioning normally, they can handle the extra protein.

3. How many carbs can you eat and still be in ketosis?

This varies based on the person, but it is generally recommended to stay below 20 net carbs each day. This can be adjusted some, up to 50 daily for those with a regular exercise routine, while remaining in ketosis. Those who are overweight or insulin-resistant will need to stick with the 20 grams of carbs daily to maintain ketosis.

4. Can you be in ketosis and still not lose any weight?

It is possible to enter ketosis and maintain it without losing weight. This is not a common occurrence but is possible. Make sure you stick with the diet and include a regular exercise routine to get your body burning fat.

5. How long does it take to enter ketosis?

Every person is different, but ketosis typically takes between two days to over a week. Those who were already eating fewer carbs will enter ketosis faster than others.

6. Can I eat fruit on Keto?

While most consider fruits healthy, they are high in sugar and carbs. This is why there are very few fruits included in the Keto diet. Certain berries like raspberries, strawberries, and blackberries are low carb and can be enjoyed in small amounts, but most should be avoided.

7. How long can the Keto diet be followed?

The Keto diet can be followed as long as you choose to do so. Although there are few long-term studies of people staying in ketosis for decades, those caring for people who have spent years in ketosis do not see harmful effects of it. Some will maintain ketosis for a few weeks and then add a few foods back to their diet, then go back to a strict Keto diet once again.

8. Can I do the Keto diet as a vegan or vegetarian?

A Keto diet is possible for those who do not eat meat, but it depends on the types of food they do allow in their diet. Some vegetarians, especially those that eat cheese and eggs, can follow Keto with some adjustments, though the first few days may be challenging. On the other hand, vegans may not be able to closely follow Keto because their diets are naturally high in carbohydrates which is the opposite of Keto.

9. When in ketosis, what should my ketone level be if tested?

When someone enters ketosis, levels are generally above 0.5 mmol/l.

10. What can I use to fight Keto breath?

Keto breath is well known for those on a strict low-carb diet. It is often described as a strong, almost fruity smell that is much like nail polish remover. This is caused by one of the ketone bodies, acetone. These higher acetone levels can also change the way the body smells when working out or sweating. Not all people will face this issue, and for those that do, it is usually temporary, but for those who want to battle the problem or who cannot seem to shake it, make sure you are getting enough salt and drinking plenty of fluids. It is also important to maintain good oral hygiene. Try breath fresheners to cover the Keto smell until it resolves, but if it does not, reduce the degree of ketosis. This means including a few more carbs in your diet, which may affect the effectiveness of the diet, slowing it down, but will help with the breath issue.

11. What is the difference between Keto and low-carb diets?

Keto is a low-carb diet but very strict. Keto also puts a stronger emphasis on moderating protein intake, so fat is the primary energy supply. Of course, a regular low-carb diet will put people in ketosis anyway, but Keto tweaks this to allow you to go into deeper ketosis.

12. Is supplementing with exogenous ketones helpful for weight loss?

While higher ketone levels help promote weight loss, adding MCT oil or exogenous ketones may hinder weight loss on the Keto diet. For weight loss, focus on carborestriction, getting enough protein, and using fats for satiety and taste. MCT oil or exogenous ketones are used predominantly when Keto is followed for performance reasons, not weight loss.

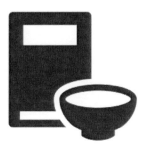

Disclaimer

This book contains opinions and ideas of the author and is meant to teach the reader informative and helpful knowledge while due care should be taken by the user in the application of the information provided. The instructions and strategies are possibly not right for every reader and there is no guarantee that they work for everyone. Using this book and implementing the information/recipes therein contained is explicitly your own responsibility and risk. This work with all its contents, does not guarantee correctness, completion, quality or correctness of the provided information. Misinformation or misprints cannot be completely eliminated.

Made in United States
North Haven, CT
17 September 2022

24236477R00067